Second Heart

"FIRST HEART BEATS FOR LOVE, SECOND HEART BEATS FOR LIFE"

Dr. Sandeep Huilgol
Santosh Avvannavar

Published by :

ARAVIND ENTERPRISES
Bengaluru

Second Heart : written by Dr. Sandeep Huilgol and Santosh Avvannavar and published by Aravind Enterprises, Bengaluru.

Copyright	:	Authors'
First Print	:	March 2014
Book Size	:	1/8th Demi
Paper Used	:	80 GSM NS Maplitho LW
Pages	:	80
Copies	:	1000
Price	:	Rs. 00/-

Published by   :   **Aravind Enterprises**
#25, 12th Main, Vijayanagar
Bengaluru 560 040
+91 9886 346 356

To shop online   :   **www.a4dable.in**

Coverpage   :   Sachin
Designed by   :   Divya Printronics, Bengaluru
Printed at   :   Lakshmi Mudranalaya

This book is dedicated to :

The Almighty God,
Parents,
Geeta Huilgol, Daughter Ananya
and Sanjay Huilgol,
Pastor Anil and Sister Glory
(New Life Fellowship Church),
In Memory of Amrita R Chandawarkar,
Raghunath Babu Are,
& Dr. Meena R Chandawarkar

Acknowledgement

We would like to thank the Almighty God for giving us ability to pen stories to glorify HIM. We thank our parents for their unconditional love and support. We thank JyothiGhiwari for the proof reading of the manuscript. We thank Ms. Lahari Basu for English to Bengali Transalation. We also thank Mr. AsharNeyaz for enriching the manuscript. We express our gratitude to our best friends Sameer Mirji, Vasudha Mirji, Amresha M, Dr. Sandeep Puranik, Dr. Santosh Hukkeri and Shrikant Managoli for being there during all the time of trials. We would also extend our gratitude to the mentors Meena R Chanda warkar, P V Ramana, N K Narasimhan; Suchita Khanna, Avinash Himanshu, Rahul Nair (motivators); Ashwin Bellur, Sujeeth Kumar and Ruchita Kumar and Dr. Sangeeta Huilgol (emotional support). We also thank Ashar Neyaz (Computer Engineer, SIT, Tumkur), Dr. Lokesh Patil (M.D.) Vineet Singh (Software Engineer at TCS), Saurav Kumar (MBA) andNithish J (Software Engineer at IBM) for constant support.

We also extend our thanks to all the reviewers (Maniparna Sengupta Majumder, Kritika Narula and others) for the novel 'Adhuri Prem Kahaniya', and 'Dear Wife, Your Husband is not a Superhero'.

We also thank Amrita Foundation for HRD (w w w . a m r i t a f o u n d a t i o n . w o r d p r e s s . c o m <http://www.amritafoundation.wordpress.com>) to allow us to pen all our thoughts since May 2012. We would like to appreciate and thank Mr. Sachin Kudturkar (Founder, Aravind India) for his patience, effort and constant inputs to bring this book out and publish on time. We wish Aravind Enterprises a great success with this second book launch. And also we thank DivyaPrintronics for their effort in making this book look elegant and beautiful.If we have missed to thank someone it could be only be accidental and not intentional. Last but not the least to all our dear students!

Dr. Sandeep Huilgol
Santosh Avvannavar

Content

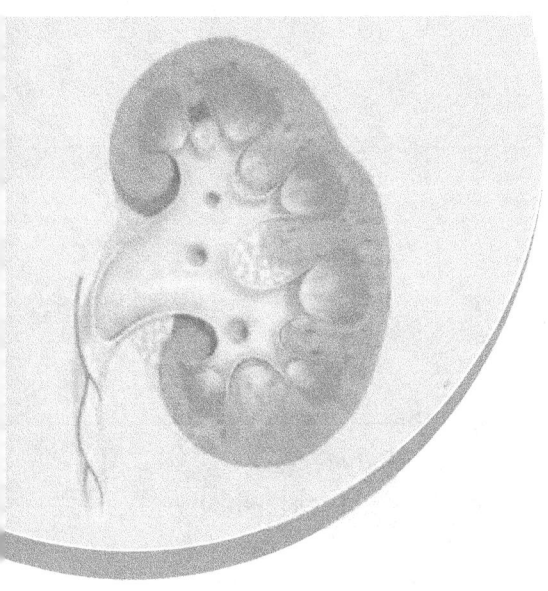

Introduction

The book encompasses five fiction stories (not interrelated) with simple narration to bring awareness about the misconceptionsassociated with kidney issues among the common people. These stories are partly based on factual stories through authors' experience. The book attempts a non-technical handling of a kidney dialysis procedural issuethrough emotive stories. Kidney diseases, although very common, people are conscious of it the least. Statistically to say about 10 percent of the general population experience some kind of kidney failure and these are the likely ones to go into a stage where they would require artificial support, which means, dialysis to replace the functions of the kidneys. Kidneys form a vital part of our body, apart from what people are aware about production of urine and removal of waste and toxic materials from the body, they regulate blood pressure and kidneys are necessary for the production of blood and supportthe proper chemical balance in the body. Even though support system for kidney failure is available (that too mostly in bigger cities), the cost of care is very huge and out of reach for the common man. Inspite of all the vital functions, they have not been able to find their due importance among the populace. With this book, the authors have tried to create awareness through stories. These characters are knitted through the use of the emotions and lighter narration style.

Love, War and Faith

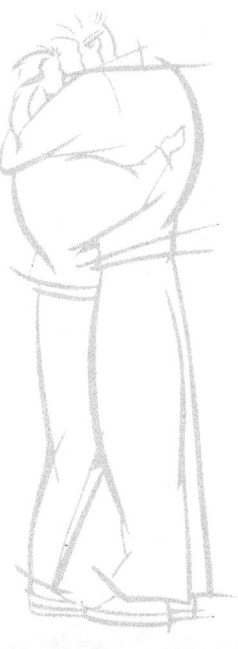

I, Priya Shankar believed that 'Life has to have all the ingredients such as romance, loving family, tragedy and happy ending.' I was always open for bold attempts such as falling in love outside our community and believed that my parents would share my opinion. Like most girls, even I had some people who admired me and perhaps happened to be in love with me. I found myself in search of someone else whom I always dreamt about to have as a life partner. I was at my aunt's place in Nainital for one-summer holidays. Two eyes were not enough to express and beautify the magnificent view of this popular hill station. I was at a coffee shop to buy a birthday cake, where I bumped into a tall, handsome man, Shankar. It wasn't something like 'Love at first sight.' I went on to invite all the children in the neighborhood for my birthday celebrations. I didn't even think Shankar would end up being a neighborhood child too. There were smiles exchanged while remembering of the Café shop's bumper while buying my birthday cake. There were neighbors' children, one elder citizen (Aunt) and one young citizen (Shankar) for my birthday celebration.

Though it was a casual meet, I found it to be chosen by my destiny. I unobtrusively observed him under a variety of circumstances and had found out all that I could about him. Love for him grew gradually in my heart. This calm and steady progression from a casual meet to love was worth a journey. I wouldn't deny if there was any physical attraction. We never asked each other to be lovebirds. It was out of choice and will to meet. We wanted to get a realistic picture of ourselves, some kinds of idealization that is expected. I was a no-no for blind romantic infatuation. I can say that we did date, but never petted. Both of us had pure desires. We were considerate and genuine for our welfare. I tried to test his intentions by inviting him to come over for lunch, whilemyaunt was offto work. He showed no desire to exploit me in any way for his personal gain. My summer vacation went unnoticed and we had to depart from the station. I was seated at thewindow to wave goodbye and he was on the platform for a cheerful goodbye. The train'ssiren went off; Shankar uttered this line 'I have lit the lamp of love with you, to turnour future brighter.' My moistened glittered eyes and bright smile werethe answer. Some circumstances kept us apart for a long time, but our love did not wane. It only deepened with time and distance. Parental objections and sharp cultural differences didn't stop us, as we thought love could overcome everything with time. "When love is not made of any religion, why should love be measured with any religion?"

I patiently waited for some vacation, and especially summer for a much-desired Nainital visit. I didn't expect that this summer would be so warm that it would bring any twist to our lives. Shankar was on leave duringthe month of April 1999. He waited at the railway station to receive me. This was perhaps the first time I hugged him, shyly. Shankar took me to his favorite spot 'NainiJheel' in Nainital; he heldmy hand, looked into my eyes said, "Let's Marry." My pulse rate was definitely high during this time andduring such an excitement the overproduction of adrenaline causes theheart to pump faster.

On the way backhome, Shankar received a message on

Second Heart

his pager, asking him to immediately call someone. He was ordered to cut short his leave to get back to the front-line of the war. Shankar tried hard to console me with a promise to return, but I was unable to take this sudden fear of losing him. Irrespective of his return(hope is good, but can become unhelpful as well) from the war at the border, I desired to have his generation to continue. He wasn't ready to do this without official marriage. This emotional moment drew us to make love that night. The next day morning he had to leave for the war and I lived in aperpetual fear for the next three weeks. He had to walk a distance and wait for the phone booth during his unoccupied time to call me. On April 15th, I heard on the radio about Shankar's death while he and other soldiers were trying to capture the post. "Do I salute and cheer for his sacrifice?" In a few days his body was brought to his village, all the people of the village were gathered near his house. I sat near his dead body, cuddling and crying loudly. His family members asked me, 'Who am I?' I kept crying louder and louder. In shrill voice I screamed, 'I am his wife'. His family didn't accept this fact and Iwas asked to leave right away. Through our family disapproved of our love and news of me becoming a mother (May 1999), I went ahead to bring our children to the world.

I moved to Bangalore in June 1999 with the help of a friend Prasoon. Within the next two weeks, with God's grace I got a job in a BPO referred by Prasoon. All looked well until July end,buton July 31st midnight, I experienced breathlessness, tiredness and was stressed out. My colleagues and Prasoon immediately rushed me to a nearbyclinic. The doctor was of the opinion that stress can often cause this because of working in the night shifts. Nonetheless, the doctor wanted to make sure that everything was alright and went on to advice for a further check-up the next day at the hospital. Other colleagues agreed with the doctor's perspective of being under stress and things would be perfectly alright after some rest. Prasoon wanted to stay with me to help me out. I was afraid of the emotional connection between us and never wanted to misguide Prasoon for his help and affection. I reminded myself of being married to Shankar and now a widow. Assured him with a promise to call him first in case need arises. I felt alright and later failed to visit the doctor. On August 15th, 1999, at the office, we were celebrating India's Independence Day with a patriotic movie screened 'Border' post the lunch. As the movie progressed, it reminded me of Shankar's face in all the soldiers. One of them being killed in the war bestowed me with a feeling of Shankar being killed in the war. I shrieked, Shankar, Shankar... breathless... I was rushed toa hospital, several medical examinations were done to reveal that there was no fetal cardiac activity and hence the pregnancy had to be terminated. I couldn't accept the fact that Shankar's child will never see a light; only a mother can understand this cry and travail of losing a child.

I went for a regular checkup with my previous medical history and reports. One of the reports (during 1997), when I was following up with a doctor for my thyroid issue (which is quite common in women) had mentioned ofmy kidneys' leaking proteins. I had ignored it in spite of doctors' advice for further follow-ups. I felt it never created any problem for me. The doctor had told me that I had a kidney issue, but I thought

Second Heart

since I do not have any problems pertaining to the urine. I had ignored it. I had taken some native medicines and never bothered about the kidneys' leaking proteins. Doctor exclaimed that. 'I may have to undergo kidney dialysis untilsurvival.' Some tests were done and few more tests, which included a kidney biopsy, took a while to get reported since the only Nephro-pathologist (a doctor who gets to know looking at the microscope and diagnosing kidney diseases) in the whole of state was on leave. I was informed that I have 'active lupus'. It's a rare form of the disease that affects most of the organs of the body. It's a disease in which the soldiers (cells) who protect our body from inside turn traitors and fight against our individual cells and organs. I was offered some treatment, but I was given less chance of recovery since most of the changes on the biopsy were irreversible, which meant my kidney damage to extent that they were not repairable. Had I taken the aforementioned doctor seriously and got myself treated I would probably have saved Shankar's child.

Back home, I was feeling really depressed. I did see myself the mirror, exclaiming in dismay at my state of life. Then, there was a doorbell and Prasoon was at the door. Seeing me in pain, he hugged me tightly. I broke down like a child in his arms. 'Why did this happen to me?', 'Why was Shankar taken away from me?', and many other unanswerable questions that spurge through my shattered heart. In succeeding few days, Prasoon proposed to marry me but I politely wished him a wonderful life with someone else. I told him to get married to someone else. I promised him to be a member of his celebrations.

I moved to Mumbai in 2001 to another BPO company to spend my remaining life and help women who have kidney diseases. Life looked good being active at work and helping others until the next seven years. The year 2008 will remain highlighted in the IT history because various people went astray due to recession. Like others, I too lost my job. I was over experienced to get a call for the job in the market in those days. I stopped going regularly for kidney dialysis as survival had become difficult with odd jobs (worked on daily or weekly wages at sometime). It was more than two years, unable to get a right job; I decided to move back to Bengaluru (was spelled Bangalore earlier). I didn't have anyone else other than Prasoon to ask for help. Prasoon was always there on the footboard to help; now his beautiful wife, Lahari and a child were part of his family. Prasoon on hearing the last one and half years'story, took me to a nephrologist. Numerous medical examinations (which cost more than a lakh rupee) were done to identify the situations those were critical. By this time, I was unable to do routine activities on my own. I had developed heart problems, my body was swollen, and lungs were filled with water, all this because I couldn't undergo the regular treatment. The condition was critical in the next few days because I had 'active lupus' with infection. Doctors were uncertain if I would survive and were actually surprised that I survived for the past nine year'sin spiteofregular treatment, this is often uncommon to survive in such complex situation. Initially the company where I worked covered my health insurance and I could get a regular treatment which made me live longer, but recession made it was difficult to manage

Second Heart

twenty thousand rupees a month for dialysis and other medications.

Today I will be moving to ventilator (artificial respirator) as I am finding it too difficult to breathe.I have an urge that others are made aware of sufferings of kidney diseases hence an author is requested to hear my story from Prasoon and my daily diary could bring awareness to millions of people about the implications of kidney diseases. While I was young, my Papa always used to tell me 'Health is wealth'. I wish I had listened to him. Prasoon will be seated next to me with a hope to see my eyes open, as I close my eyes eternally. His wife would be on fast for my speedy recovery or ask God to give me some place in heaven. His child would be wondering, why Aunty is not talking or playing with him? By the time you read this story, I would have left this world.

Doctor's diary:

Often it is realized that patients do not take the advice given by a Doctor seriouslyand some unfortunate among thempay a heavy price for that. Various times people resort to alternative medications that are also associated with toxic to the kidneys. Priya Shankar in the story had ignored the doctor's advice to undergo further evaluation after she was found to have protein leakage into the urine and she took some alternative treatment. Had she seen a specialist doctor at that time, probably she would not have suffered so much.

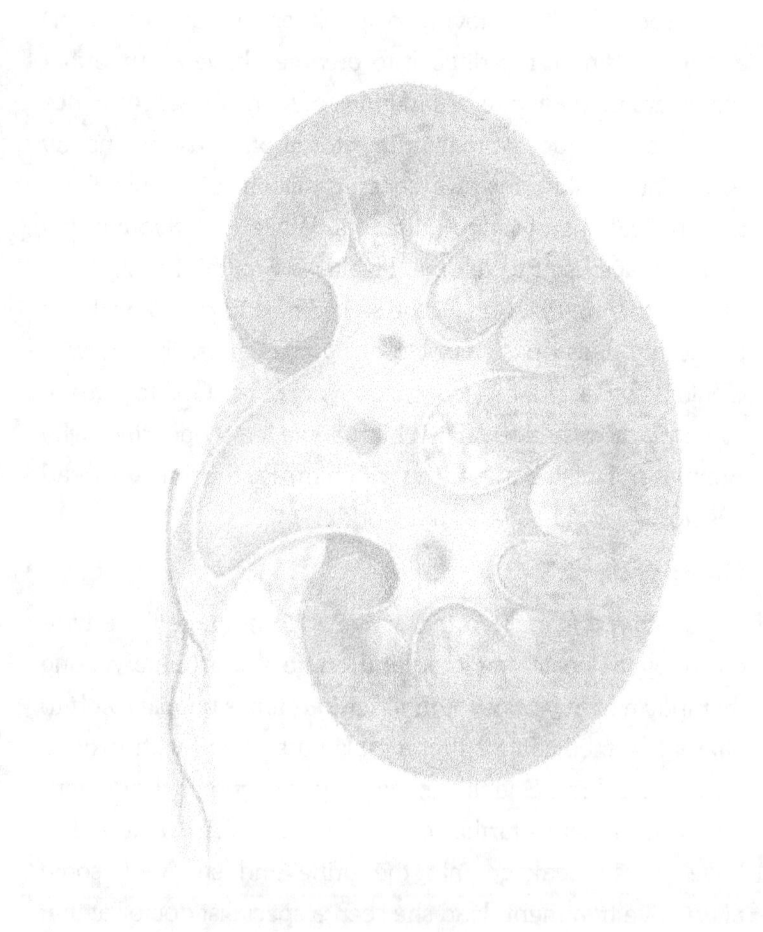

Hope

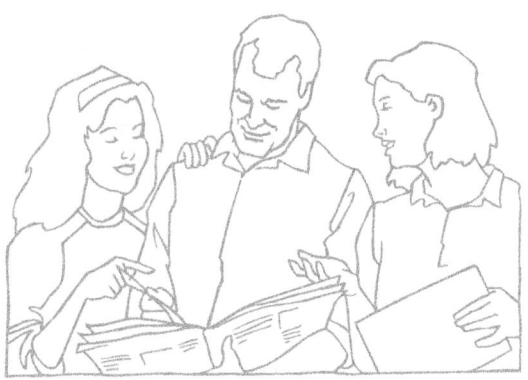

Hope neither has a beginning nor an end; it is complete within itself. Before anything (space, time or physical matter) love and hope existed. Hope and love are perfect in every way and are not limited in anyway. Do these two things bring purpose to one's life in this world? Do these two things have a purpose beyond this world? Those, who seek answers and are listening, there is 'Hope and Love'.

It is around six in the morning. The weather is quite cold. It is about 16 degree Celsius. The hospital is still inactive. The registration area is still not open on the ground floor. There are few patients here and there in the waiting area on the ground floor. A lot of patients, some in the wheelchair, some accompanied by their wives or children are all rushing to the lift. All seem to know each other very well. The new patients to the hospital were prettyinquisitive seeing all this. An old Hyderabadi asked a security guard, "Kahanjaaraheyhai ye sab logaa?"(Where are these people going?). The security guard, busy arranging all the chairs (did not even lift his head) replied, "Chacha sixth floor."

Somewhere on the sixth floor of the building, on the east wing, there is a dialysis unit. As soon, as you get out of the lift and walk a few steps on the right there is a reception area of the dialysis unit. Uma, the young receptionist (wearing a red saree with a gilt border, and a blouse, matching that) sits in front of one of the computers, and register the patients coming to the dialysis. There is a lounge area, where patients along with their guardians wait before being called inside the dialysis unit for their turn. There are three shifts for patients everyday starting at 7 am, four hours each session and one hour gap in between to clean the dialysis machine. The same machine is used for the patient in the next shift.

I (Young Geetha, that's how people here address me) am waiting alone for my turn. I come from some place in the northern part of the country; have travelled about 1500 kilometers to this hospital, as I could not get any facility near my place. Now I have rented a room with all the elementary facilities. I am told that I need a few days of dialysis and my kidneys may recover. I do not know, what to do in case they don't? I get shivers down my spine thinking hereafter. In case, I need a long-term medical treatment what will I do?

As soon as we enter the dialysis area there are about 25 machines. They are basically pumping machines that draw blood from our body and pass it through a filter fitted to it and give it back to the body and in the process cleansing the blood from all the impurities. Each dialysis machine has a chair or a bed by the side of it and Uma allocates us to a particular machine.

It's a safe and good place to be. All the patients know each other and they spend most of their time with the other patients. They are all like one giant family, consisting of patients, dialysis nurses and their guardians.

Selvam and me: November 8th 2013

AbhayKumar: Good Morning Shashidhar and Young Geetha.

Shashidhar: Good Morning to you as well.

Me:	Gooood Morning … Abhay.
AbhayKumar:	Where is Mr. Selvam? I have seen his dialysis bay empty since few sessions.
Me:	Who is Mr. Selvam?
AbhayKumar:	Selvam, he has been regularly irregular for the dialysis room.
Shashidhar:	Selvamhas been my patient for one year. He was in the military, lost his leg during firing at the border in 2011. He comes from Krishnagiri, Tamil Nadu with two daughters aged 10 and 12.
Me:	I like people from the army. They have a great physique. What happened to his wife?
Shashidhar:	Unfortunately, he lost her in an accident two years ago.
Me:	Oh, sorry to hear that. (On a lighter note) I am still young and single (38 years old) to mingle with the solider.
Shashidhar:	Oh ho! He took voluntary retirement at the age of 40 after he lost his wife. He has a pension of 5000 (Five Thousand Rupees). His house rent is 1000 (One Thousand Rupees), spends about 2000 (Two Thousand Rupees) for a monthly travel to the dialysis unit. He is lucky to be covered under the ex-servicemen beneficiary

scheme of government; otherwise he would have never made it to the dialysis unit.

AbhayKumar: I always enjoyed tales of war narrated by Selvam.

Me: I have been visiting the dialysis room only since two weeks. Doctors have told my kidney functions might recover and it would be a temporary dialysis. I do not know many people in this unit. Where is Selvam?

Shashidhar: I work in this hospital as a staff nurse. I get to know all their stories as many of them share their personal stories as well. He has a lot of difficulties managing family with the pension he gets. I remember one day there was a bus strike; he slept in our hospital garden for two days to take the alternate day's dialysis. He wanted to admit his children in a boarding school so that his children are looked after in case he dies. He spent all his savings for this purpose and got them admitted to an orphan boarding school in Kerala. Today he lies in the emergency ward and has difficulty in breathing owing to irregular dialysis.

Me: I am willing to help Selvam for his dialysis. Shashidhar, can you take Abhay and me to the emergency ward after our dialysis?

Second Heart

Shashidhar:	That's really nice of you. Yes, definitely! I will.
Me:	I am excited to see Mr. Selvam.
AbhayKumar:	It's an emergency ward, not a make-up room.
Me:	(Smiled!)

Abhay and me along with Shashidhar rushed to the emergency ward to see Mr. Selvam. He was brought dead outside the emergency ward on a stretcher. Abhay's heart sank with a thought. "Will I also be in the same state very soon?"

Abhay and me: November10th 2013

Shashidhar:	Good Morning Geetha....Oops Young Geetha
Me:	(stared at Shashidhar,Abhay and appeared lost. My mind was numb)
Shashidhar:	What's the matter with Young Geetha?
Me:	I feel guilty for being unable to help Selvam. Such a handsome man, he was just 40 years old.
AbhayKumar:	Handsome...Young...hmm (Here is young, 34 year old handsome lying next to her, and she worries about dead-says in his mind)
Me:	Why someone couldn't help him?
AbhayKumar:	Help! What kind?

Me:	Donate a kidney or give some money for dialysis.
Shashidhar:	You should hear from Abhay an interesting story about organ donation.
Me:	Smiles, Abhay, please tell me the story.
AbhayKumar:	You promise to 'Marry Me' after listening to my story. (He giggles)
Me:	Abhaay…!
AbhayKumar:	Alright!
AbhayKumar:	I joined a family run business, after an MBA.
Me:	Another MBA moron!
AbhayKumar:	Yes, a big moron!
Me:	Sorry for being so spontaneous. Abhay continue with your story. I will lock my lips until you complete the story.
AbhayKumar:	Alright! About eight years ago, I was identified with kidney failure. We ran various advertisements requesting for an altruistic donor (One who donates an organ through free will). After a month wait, one person came forward to donate but neededsome security for his family and we agreed to all his terms to motivate him to donate.
Me:	That's an entirely altruistic act he hehe,

Second Heart

......(in a sarcasticway). I questioned, how altruistic his motives were?

AbhayKumar: Inspite fulfilling all the promises, he backed out.

Me: Why did he back out?

AbhayKumar: That's quite difficult to answer, but there could be many reasons for it.

Me: What kind of reasons?

AbhayKumar: Hmm... misconceptions such as one cannot survive with one kidney or health complications that could occur on donation.

Me: Even I didn't know one could survive with only one kidney.

AbhayKumar: Not only kidney, a person has a choice to donate eyes, skin, heart, liver and othersafter one's death, especially brain death. Relatives just have to agree to donate organs of their loved ones after their death. People in need of any organ should register in the government 'cadaver donation program' through a nephrologist and other specialists in any major hospitals. Each state has its specific model of donation and different rules.

Me: Oh, 'A Corpse Donation Program', you are aware a lot about all this.

AbhayKumar:	Smiles, I can almost write a thesis on transplant and have been struggling for getting myself a kidney. I know a lot of nuances about transplantation, legal procedures and some aspects of medical procedures as well. I did register myself three years ago as a recipient but am very low in the transplant waiting list.
Me:	I heard one might die at a chronic stage (kidney failure). How are you alive? Sorry to be rude.
AbhayKumar:	Don't be sorry for your curiosity. My family came forward to donate the kidney and thankful to them for this. My wife's blood group didn't match though there was a possibility it was difficult to afford the complex operations. My mother being a diabetic patient, her kidney donation was out of the question but was fortunate enough to have father's kidney.
Me:	Wow, that's nice! Why should you be still undergoing dialysis?
AbhayKumar:	Unfortunately, the replaced kidney was rejected very soon.
Me:	Oh, I am sorry! Why doesn't the government takes care of this?
AbhayKumar:	What should the government do? They have many schemes, but people are afraid

Second Heart

to come forward to donate. People are not motivated enough to donate organs, even after death. *Cadaver donation* generates a huge number of organs in many developed countries that can give a new life to someone in need and in some countries infact *cadaver donation* is compulsory.

Me: I mean, the government can serve as mediators between donors and recipients. Some security from recipients to donor's family and this could be a good motivation to donate.

AbhayKumar: Exactly!!! Yes, some countries have legalized the system of organ donation. I mean a kind of selling. A Government body or an NGO acts as a mediator between the donor and recipient to make sure the donor is properly compensated.

Look my logic is, I amin needof a kidney and someone somewhere is in need of money for his livelihood. Why not both of us get benefited?

Me: Oh! I forgot I am talking to a businessman. (Smiles)

AbhayKumar: See the poor man will continue to be poor most of the time and his generations to come may continue to be in the same situation, so rather an NGO can intervene and strike a deal between both the parties, instead of direct financial exchange. The recipient can take care of his children's education, health and medical expenses.

Me: Challenges exist. But the Government should think a way out.

AbhayKumar: Let's hope at least a future generations gets this opportunity.

Me: Abhay, I shall donate my kidney in case they recover and if you promise to marry me.

AbhayKumar: Smiles and laughs!

Aryan and me: November 13ᵗʰ 2013

Shashidhar: Good Morning Young Geetha! Good Morning Abhay!

Abhay Kumar and me: (Smiles at Shashidhar)

Me: I see a young (12 years old) boy in the corner since a week. Shashidhar, who is he?

Shashidhar: He is Aryan, undergoing dialysis since a week. He has poor flow of urine leading to accumulation of urine in the bladder and causing *reflux*.

Me: Care to explain Shashidhar…

Shashidhar: It is something similar to backwaters. Whenever a dam is built across a river, the backwaters can flood causing destruction of so many villages, property and all. It is something akin to that. Reflux of urine will damage the kidneys. This was seen at the age of three in Aryan. He had a poor stream of urine, but elders in the family neglected it thinking it's a common phenomenon. In reality, his mother says that a doctor had advised them that he needs treatment, which would be a minor surgery, but they ignored listening to elders who are supposed to be more experienced with dozens of children.

Me: Poor child.

Shashidhar: Yes a poor child.

AbhayKumar: He is lucky to have a financial donor, but Selvam was very unlucky in this matter.

Me: Who is that great person?

Shashidhar: In 2006, we had a patient in our hospital. The owner of a large chain of restaurants in Mumbai was suffering from diabetes. Dr. Sameer advised him to have regular follow-up on. He was very regular for the first six months later got himself too much occupied as business grew. We did send him many reminders as a part of follow-up, but he hardly turned up. Diabetes as you know is a killer disease if neglected. Infact, diabetes is the leading cause of kidney disease in India, for that matter in the world. In 2010 he was brought to our hospital in a very critical condition (breathing difficulty) and he was declared dead in the emergency ward. Being rich and educated, but non-compliant with doctors' advice, which cost him his life. After this incident, his family decided to help one patient every year.

Me: I have now come to know a lot about kidney diseases in the last few days. I am feeling I should do anything for the kidney patients.

(Dr. Sameer enters the dialysis unit for a routine round)

Dr. Sameer: Geetha, you are a teacher isn't it?

Me: Yes, Doc. I am a teacher. Although I may not earn much, my dad is rich and I am the only child. I can help monetarily with the help of my dad.

Dr. Sameer: Geetha, you are so sweet. God bless!!Nevertheless, I won't ask for monetary help but see, you all very well know that, "Prevention is better than cure". Why not do your bits by educating your students? You can bring a lot of changes by educating about kidney diseases. Now

	people are very much consciousabout HIV and that has made a lot of difference.
AbhayKumar:	Doctor, people are worried so much about basic needs, why would they be interested in something very rare?
Me:	I was about to ask the similar question. Doctor, how widespread is kidney disease?
Dr. Sameer:	You will be worried and surprised to know the prevalence of kidney diseases is about 10% in the general population.
Me:	Oh no!! That's a huge number…
AbhayKumar:	Doctor you mean to say in 100 crore populations, 10 crorehave kidney disease. That's a lie, isn't it?
Dr. Sameer:	No Abhay, that's exactly the number. 10% of people will get some form of kidney disease. Not all may lead to end stage disease where they land up in dialysis. However, these are the people at risk.
AbhayKumar:	Oh, okay.
Dr. Sameer:	And the rest you know. Once someone reaches a stage where dialysis is required,it's somewhere up to twenty thousand rupees a month based on the hospital and medication costs extra. Apart from this, they need to visit the dialysis unit thrice a weekand time, energy, money spent on the

	dialysis visit does often cost more. It's a geometric progression.
Me:	And the dialysis facilities are also not there in smaller places, even if you can afford, you don't have the facility to undergo dialysis.
AbhayKumar:	And you know Geetha, the number of nephrologists in the country. For such a huge number of patients,there only about 1500 Nephrologists!!
Dr. Sameer:	Yeah, you are right Abhay.
	(There is a prolonged silence after this. Everyone is lost in some thought)
Dr. Sameer:	Goodbye Geetha, bye Abhay........ Shashi, any other problematic patient? You had called me for some flow, issues of some patient. I forgot about that and was lost in this conversation.
Shashidhar:	She is there in the corner bed doctor (He points to the old woman*Balliamma* in the left hand corner towards the reuse area).
	(And they both hurry towards that....)

Doctor's diary:

Diabetes is the most common cause of kidney diseases in the world and it often leads to thefinal point of renal failure if neglected and dialysis, becomes imperative to survive. Once someone is on dialysis the expenses are manifold. Dialysis costs about 15 to 30 thousand a month depending on the unit, apart from this the person undergoing dialysis will have to invest a lot of time coming to the dialysis unit, spending time on the machine for four hours thrice a week. The cost of medicines when someone arrives at this stage of the disease adds up and most importantly the person is immune-compromised and prone to infections and repeated hospitalizations adding to the cost of care. Never ignore diabetes; strict control, diet modification, lifestyle changes and exercisesare must. Strictly follow doctors advise on treatment and have a proper, systematic follow-up.

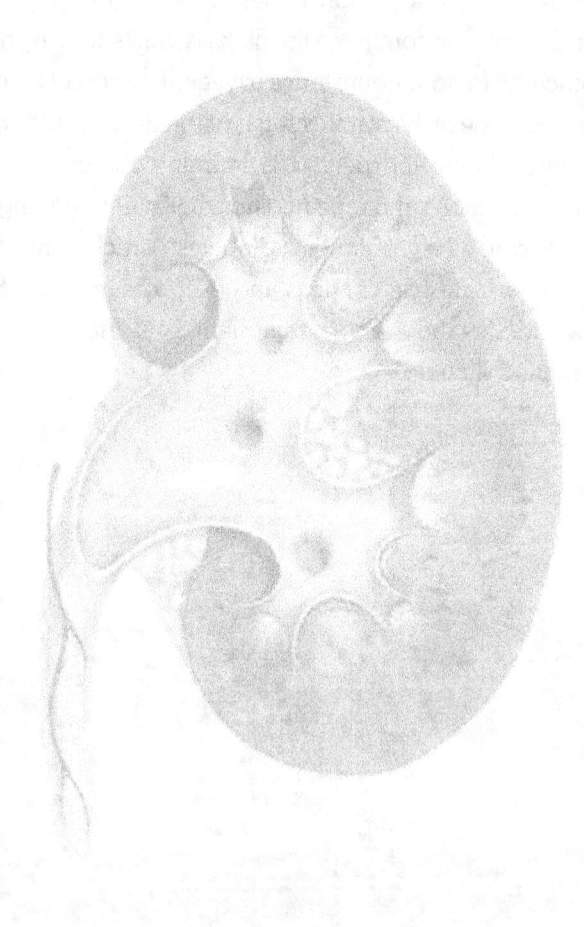

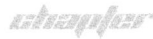

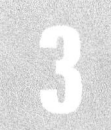

3

Unforgotten Love, Love That Returned & Faith

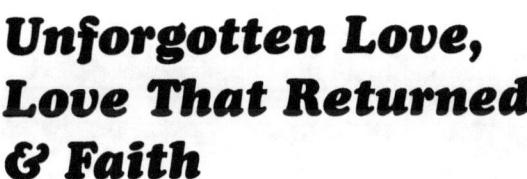

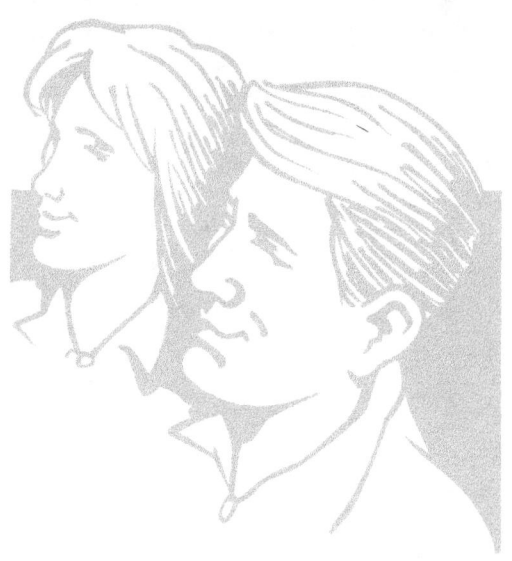

There are mainly (mostly) two things Indian parents aspire (the dream) fortheir children Engineer and/or Doctor. I am alsoa victim of this system and was forced to become a doctor. I though hated the idea of being a doctor, fiddle with corpses initially and be a living corpse later. My parents were no less in coloring a brighter picture of the future in comparison with my friends that opted commerce, arts and music.

I always wondered, how lucky bastards my friends were to get a girlfriend at the age of 19, have all the fun until 23! I was living in a campus of 30:1 of boys: girls ratio. Even that '1', the seniors pursuing post-graduation took away, as it brought security to a girl and her family. By the time she graduated, he would have done with most desired master's courses like M.S or M.D. My wait to become three years senior in a medical college gave a bald head. I had to forget the thought of a girl; even women won't look at me.

For practical's, Dr.VichitraGundamani (Incharge faculty) had split us into groups of eight. There was this one soul (girl, Swati) who was a part of our group, a girl who had oily hair with hair drawn back and tied like a ponytail and thick eyeglasses. I wished to take a ride across the college holding that lovely ponytail. She would often see me and shy away. My friends in the group would say, Bhai ladki line derahihai (brother, she's giving you mixed signals'). I was more interested in the neighboring girls from an engineering college adjacent to the medical college.

During the first year of laboratory studies (practical) every other student acted like a patient (specimen) to help the

Second Heart

other teammates learn. Swati was checking my Blood Pressure; it gave a high reading (quite unusual). She made fun of me saying, 'I am hot and your blood is boiling.' Dr. Vichitra was of the opinion that it may be due to stress of long study hours. Only doctors and engineers can tell how time flies by during undergraduation. I did find a girlfriend (Tina) from the neighboring engineering college, but the relationship ran into trouble within a few months because of the '**Ten Commandments**' to date medical students

- We are rarely to be seen. Ever.

- We always have great affairs. Books are our first girl/boy friends. Unfortunately!

- We always talk about functioning of the body during a date.

- We often fail in the class tests, cry like a baby initially and laugh like the joker rest of our lives.

- We have new illnesses ranging from rare to mundane. If someone dates us, they become one (ill) because of this union.

- We are highly liable to make anyone feel that 'you don't have a boyfriend.'

- We remind, alert and command our girlfriends of the germs and infectious diseases.

- We date like commercial ads for a few minutes. Preferably during lunch break of twenty-five minutes. It's not thirty minutes because five minutes are needed to walk back from the entrance of the

Second Heart

college. Yes, we date at the entrance of the college in the open.

- It's not uncommon to be in a library and hooked on books for eight to ten hours a day, as we need to know all the diseases that had existed and likely to exist if the earth continues to survive.

- We don't know if there are birthdays, anniversaries and sometimes get as far as forgetting the birth of our own first-born.

She tried hard to bear with me for the last two years, but I was helpless because medical college completely consumed me. I was in the final year of studies when she joined as a software engineer in a multinational IT company. We tried to keep in touch, but the distance mattered for her and it was never the same. I would think about her, smile a minute when I came across something that reminded me of her. I was sure to make this relationship work by closing in on the infinite-seeming distance that was keeping us apart. Just a few months before the closure year of education, I received a note from the Dean of the medical school stating that I would be the best outgoing student; only topper of the college used to receive it. I arranged a surprise date (can you imagine a medical student doing such a thing?) for Tina at her favorite place and she was delighted at the surprise!

I opened the Champagne as a symbol of success, love and a new beginning and saw a dazzling smile on her face. I bowed down on my knee, took a ring, held left hand of hers to put the ring saying, "I love you" and "Together Forever". All of a sudden I felt very difficult to breathe, collapsed and fell on the ground.

I opened my eyes after a few hours in an emergency ward of a hospital; Tina was seated at a distance and my family members in tears. Medical reports declared that the kidneys aren't functioning and have to be put for the regular dialysis. My health history reminded me of the unusual B.P. record in the 1st year of MBBS. I used to get tired unusually, but I used to attribute to the stress related to studies, especially in the final year of medical college and that negligence has cost a lot. Afterwards, I discovered that most of the kidney diseases are without symptoms until it reaches a point where it is not reversible and can only be found out with regular and reliable health checkup. Atleast I had a warning of high blood pressure, which wasneglected. Even on that particular day in the morning I felt a bit breathless, but that I thought because of the cold weather. Do I have to pay more for that negligence? Tina left me alone due to her family pressure.I felt like being court marshaled and declared a traitor. With a heavy heart, I moved to my hometown after graduation. Since then, I am on dialysis. Moved to Bengaluru, as it was difficult to find doctors in and around my hometown for the dialysis. My mother came forward to donate her kidney and the transplant was successful.

It's been three years married to Swati. Although this started with no feelings towards her, but eventually we fell in love with each other. I work at a hospital in assisting nephrologists, as one's own experience can help others and I had developed an interest to work and help kidney patients.

Second Heart

I received a call from the receptionist to attend a patient in the emergency ward kept in a different room. I saw a beautiful lady lying with hair fallen on her face. I tried to adjust the posture and hair and to my shock, it was Tina. I was numb and sat quietly near her with tears rolling down my cheeks. Her medical reports revealed that she has acute kidney failure. She had lost her husband in an accident; the accident was severe enough that she had lost her kidney functions owing to blood loss and low blood pressure (hypotension).

Kidneys are peculiar organs and very imperative to the functioning of our body. They are like a filter, which removes all the noxious substances generated as a by-product during body metabolism. They maintain water and acid base balance in the body and most importantly regulate the blood pressure. Despite the fact thatthe heart pumps the blood to the body, it's the kidneys, which regulate the blood pressure. Kidneys require almost 25% of the absolute blood supply. Any small fall in blood pressure due to various reasons be it blood loss because of any reason or dehydration due to anything as seemingly minor as loose motion, even heavy exercise, sunstroke and others can causea temporary shutdown of the kidneys that is recoverable, but if this prolongs which can lead to permanent renal failure.

After a few hours, she was conscious. Even she was surprised to see me subsequent to her. She was unable to have an eye contact owing to the guilt. I had already forgotten and forgiven about the past. In our talk, she learnt that Suresh (my elder brother) couldn't get married, as each and every proposal considered kidney disease is hereditary, which is in fact not true. Unfortunately, we could never find a bride for him. She felt disheartened on knowing this. My family members came to see her. Suresh decided to be an altruistic donor to Tina in case her kidney functions don't recover. My family members have seen me struggling with kidney disease and everyone has slowly developed a soft corner towards people with kidney failure. It was no less than a Shahrukh movie, an emotional drama. Each one of us was hugging, crying, smiling, and laughing with a new hope to live. Have faith to open your eyes, be sure to open both eyes to accept, appreciate and give others.

Doctor's diary:

Many a times kidney diseasesare diagnosed incidentally. There are certain warning signs, which should not be overlooked. Like our protagonist, in the above story he was found to have high blood pressure, which he ignored, and that can happen with medical professionals as well. He finally ended up in the last stage of renal failure where he required dialysis. He also had a weakness, swelling of face occasionally, which he ignored. Certain warning signs, which should not be ignored areuntimely high blood pressure, blood in the urine, weakness in the legs or face swelling. They may warrant kidney disease and if it is still in a nascent stage, either it can be treated or it can be controlled.

Second Heart

God, Freewill, and Lucifer : Battle Ground

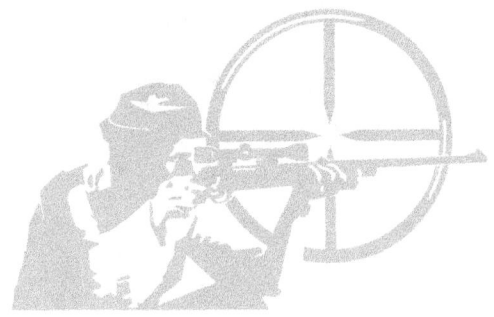

Aspirations, dreams and career are worthy, but these struggles of chasing our dreams can cost a fortune. I, Neha Jacob, got lost in the midst of a multicoloredworld, forgot that it's a God's creation. Self (desires of Satan) had come before the God, F-l-e-s'**H**' (Flesh) before 'Him'. Jacob (my husband) deep down in his heart knew this relationship would never work! I was always fascinated by things he said to me 'not' to do. Do not smoke, no alcohol, no premarital sex and so on. Today I admit that those 'not' commands were given out of his love and wisdom to help me avoid the unfavorable results. I admit this because it has costed more than desired and I embarrassed Jacob all the time. Perhaps this 'Eve' nature has existed since the creation of the earth by God. The battle of good (God), and evil (Lucifer) through us (Man) with a gift of free will (Choices) will continue until man learns to defeat the Satan (the Evil Spirit) through God.

Jacob exercised his authority and domination over my acts always, but I was unable to give a nod to his preaching's because of my selfish desires. Those selfish desires (money, career growth, worldly things), and undemanding nature of Jacob, marriage was like a convenience to me. I often threatened him to divorce or register a complaint of harassment in case he overpowers me. He did not withdraw his love; I separated myself from him through my personal choice. My spirit and soul had parted, making my mind completely dysfunctional.

I loved skyscrapers, glitzy and opulent world of fashion. Whenever I was bored, I would think "I would do my private thing today by taking off for somethingexciting, go somewhere scintillating or meet someone provocative that I'm not supposed to". I was late most (all) nights, would tell Jacob about my need to let off a little steam. I would always blame him for my behavior for being late back home and drinking a glass. I am sure like me many play these little games. Jacob would sit quiet and go back into prayers.

I was still in search and need of a happening place. I would always check out for another man and buy a drink for him and he would be smiling forconsiderable time at me for that drink. I would roll my fingers to ask and say, "Hello. What's up? I'll bet you I could score tonight, if I wanted to". In spite of the incessant reminders of being married, I preferred not to consider it. I fell for the age-old temptation game. This pre-divorce game seemed to never end until and unless it hit me unbearably one day. The fear, guilt, shame, rebellion, pride, rejection, lethargy, broken bondage, adultery and lust hit so badly that it seemedunreasonable.

Painkiller medicines for headache (stress) had become regular due to my imbalanced life. I treated Jacob as a piece of ATM (All Time Money) and a sex toy. I would feel fatigued quite often and painkillers were the solution. Once I developed a severe headache and stiff neck pain, asked Jacob, to give painkiller from the drawer. He was reluctant to give. Instead, insisted check and see a doctor right away. I collapsed unconscious between these arguments. Jacob took me to Dr. Rita, who heard our complete story from Jacob, who was broken and depressed.

Dr. Rita called us to discuss the medical report after two days. I saw Jacob worried and concerned; my heart sank for the first time for him. Dr. Rita mentioned to us in the talk that I have 'Subarachnoid Hemorrhage' a very serious condition that occurs owing to bursting of small blood vessels on the surface of the brain. This often can happen owing to hypertension, smoking and excessive alcohol intake. 40% of hospitalized patients suffer an average mortality (death) rate of 40% in the first month. This meant to have only 30 days to live together. I became sober, felt guilty and returned to Jacob's arms. Jacobalthough broken, held my hand and prayed to God. I was advised to be in the hospital (Care unit) for the ensuing 30 days; Jacob took off from his work.

Dr.Rita and her team would visit me every day with a hope that I would make it one more day. On day 2, Jacob was frantically praying and I started crying out loud repenting to Jacob. The words (God's words) that I didn't even know flowed effortlessly out of me from some source. These were the words that Jacob was longing to hear. We both started crying and that emotional moment brought us together. He held my hand and said, 'Sweet heart I have forgiven and forgotten', and 'I am confident God will.' This was the beginning of our (more of mine) true love and reconciliation of mine. Our relationship grew stronger as Jacob read scriptures to me daily and I followed his words. It was the 25th day; Dr. Rita came over to see us in the care unit. She expressed her surprise in the improvement of my health and everything seemed normal. Jacob immediately went on his knee and started to praise God for his miracle. Even this world looked undersized for the happiness of longer life. Dr. Rita asked me to commit to God that I would always remain as Jacob's love. I had become a genuine bride that day!

We went back home and later that same night I saw a dream (vision) of someone carrying away divorce papers and leave through the front door. I felt like the dejected Lucifer (Satan) ran away from my home. I eventually gave up drinking and smoking. Years passed over, with Jacob serving in a multinational IT company as a Vice-President and I am anaccomplished housewife taking care of our two children. I don't forget to say 'I love you Jacob' and thank God for making me a right person. Dr. Rita had a peaceful death last week. I received a letter from Dr. Rita during her final few days.

Dear Neha Jacob,

Greetings from me!

I hope you are doing fine. As a doctor, we ought not to be in touch with patients post the treatment. I had to go a little beyond this unsaid proclamation due to a couple of reasons. While your husband Jacob brought you to the hospital,for treatment, the hypothesis (medical reports-*Subarachnoid Hemorrhage*) was falsified over '*Acute Kidney Disease*' by me. The '*Acute Kidney Disease*' and sometimes even permanent kidney failure (renal failure) is frequently seen among various professionals owing to stress related intake of many over the counter medications including painkillers or some drugs and especially in those who are vulnerable like old aged and diabetic people. This was potentially curable in your case.

Second Heart

It often remains unresolved, and patients don't return to us owing to the free choice they adopt for second and third opinion from other doctors. This system I name it, as 'Doctor Shopping' similar to 'Window Shopping' and patientsget lost to follow-up, eventually landing at greater risk of kidney damage.That perhaps was not the right problem in your case. You might have been cured, but you were needed to get back to Jacob's life too so I set you both up! You may think how aggressive I can be! I would like to tellyou another secret; Jacob is my adopted child. He was never made aware of it, as it was my choice not to let him know about it. I hope you keep upthe secret, as one shouldn't proclaim the good deeds through the trumpet. If his actual mother was to be alive, even she would have desired what I have. I hope you will forgive me, in case hurt on learning the truth.

God bless you and your family,
Yours truly,
Rita

This letter has further strengthened my hope and faith. Her act has saved our marriage, children and family; and bestowedus a new beginning. Thank you Dr. Rita, with God all things are possible!

Doctor's diary:

Painkillers are most commonly used over the counter medications. These are quite commonly associated with kidney failure many times leading to lasting kidney failure. Somebody who is a diabetic or aged or someone who already has a milder degree of kidney damageis at higher risk. The most common scenario that specialists come acrossisan old, diabetic individual who has some or the other aches and pains, they take painkillers that are easily obtainable in any shop and land up with renal failure. Over the counter intake of some medicines should be avoided otherwise the price you pay for it might as wellbe higher.

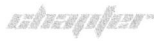

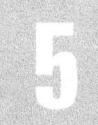

Shalom

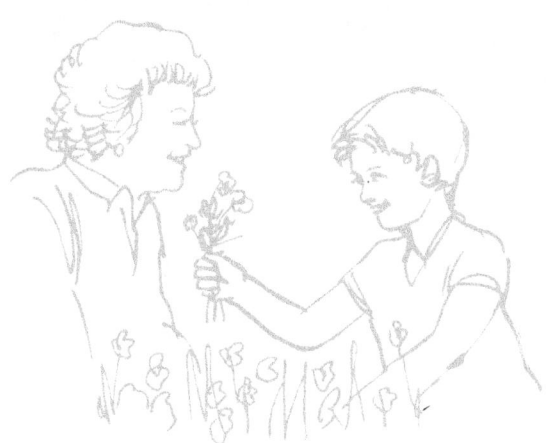

A century ago, my great grandparents settled in the colorful, vibrant, bustle and jostledcity, of Kolkata (earlier known as Calcutta) A city of Joy. I, Maya Basu,was born in 1970 during an auspicious week that is widely celebrated across the country. Ours was a big joint family (15 members) that consisted Naina (youngest sister), Aryan (elder brother), maternal and paternal parents along with cousins. Any Bengali would love to be a part of this city. This city is labeled as "The City of Palaces", "The City of processions", "The Cultural Capital of India" and "The City of Joy", but I loved the final label.

I loved some fairy tales and some true stories narrated by myGranny (grandmother) and my mother. The stories and *lullabies* (in Bengali) would send me to sleep. One of the nice little stories told by Granny(Dida in Bengali) was about the reason behind the name of 'Calcutta'. While Englishmen ruled our country, they asked one of the farmers about the name of the city. Then, the farmers did not understand English (language). The farmer thought that the Englishmen were asking, "When did you cut this paddy?" and in reply he said "Kalkatta" (cut yesterday in Hindi) and it was named as Calcutta. I grew up in this city listening to fairy tales and awaited a hero to come into my life.

Every year our whole family would go to the east bank of the river Hooghly to learn and do rituals as part of our family tradition. All the girls and women of the family wore 'TantSaree', but I preferred to wear skirts to sarees. My mother would motivate me a lot to wear 'TantSaree' and granny would

Second Heart

whisper saying 'Shona, Tomara Raja asatehabe' (Your Raja will come, baby). I would smile and ask her 'Eta kisatya' (Is it true?). 'PratisrutiShona'(promise baby) and she would giggle. I considered only married people should wear the sareehence I being single would stick to skirt and blouse. Although I used to go with the family to perform rituals, but never likedorunderstood rituals, which used to be performed just as a formality, but they were never put into practice. I would sit on the bank of the river and think of my hero (Raja) that he would come from the Far East in a boat and take me far away from these rituals. I liked the post-ritual part as it involved a visit to the Indian Museum, a Bengali movie, Travel in Human-pulled Rickshaws, Ferry Travel and Dine out at Esplanade, the heart of Calcutta. I always was waiting for this day, it gave us freedom to shop, eat and laugh openly. A day that belonged to me! The only a thing that remained as a fairy tale was 'Raja' (My Hero) came to take me away. This continued until the age of 15.

When I turned 16, an elder woman in the family insisted me wear saree everyday. I would cry and make a scene out of this every day. On the family ritual day while I was reluctant to wear saree. Granny came over to my room and said in her persuasion tone, Shona Maya 'Amar bachchaerom-korchekano?' (Why my baby is behaving like this?)

Granny:	Tomar Raja k dekhteechchakorche? (Do you like to see your Raja?)
Me:	Hya Dida (Yes Granny)
Me:	Kintugotoponerobochorshetoasheni? (But he has never come inthe last 15 years.)

Granny:	Shona, Tumitohkonodin o tant r shariporoni, kikoreashbe o? (Baby, How would he come as you never worn '*Tant Saree*'?)
Me:	Tai naki (Is it so?)
Granny:	Hya, otai (Yes it is)
Me:	O amaikothadiyeche j shariporle o nishchoiashbe (Promise that he would come if I wore saree)
Granny:	Pratisruti (Promise)

I felt as a Woman after wearing a saree. I really liked myself. My family members were pleased with thecontemporaryavatar of mine. A feeling of transformation of a girl to a woman was generated by, the way others looked at me. I was standing at some distance on the steps of the river Hooghly, a person slid over me as he missed his step over the spilt oil. We both rolled over each other until we fell into the river. My family members were shocked; Granny kept calling out for help. They were relieved as soon as we were seen over the water surface. I was very indignant, turned to slap the guy, but his charming face gave me goose bumps. 'My Raja' was here. I couldn't utter a word for the next few moments.

(We were still standing in the water)

Granny and others (stood on the first step) : Shona, tumithikacho? (Baby, are you alright!)

Me: Hya, Dida (Yes,Granny). We were mesmerized at each other.

My father pulled us out of water, gave us warm clothes to dry our hair and skin. We continued to stare at each other while drying hair and wiping wet skin.

Father: Babu, tumi Bangla jano? (Babu, Do you know Bengali?)

Babu: 'Ami khubolpo Bangla jani.' (He replied,I know very little Bengali.)

Father: Babu, tomarnaamki?(Babu, What is your name?)

Babu: Amar nam Raja. (My name is Raja.)

I felt a complete transformation from a girl to a woman on seeing Raja. He followed us at all the places. When I was onMirzaGhalib Street buying a pair of bangles,a voice came from behind-

Raja: "TumhariAankhenHumkoBulatiHai,

Par Dar Sa LagtaHaiki

ZyadaNazdeekiyaan Hone Par

BichadneKaDard Na BadhJaye"

Me: "Mirzathochalegayemagar Ghalibkoya-hinchodgaye" (Mirza has left Ghalib behind)

Raja: "Aappeneela rang acchalagtahai" (Blue color suits you)

I bought blue bangles with his affirmation. While we were at ChandniChowk, he left a note at a sweet shop counter with a nod. I nodded in affirmation to his action. I picked the note from the shop that had a short message-

"SitaronkiRoshniekUmmeedDetiHaiki

Hum Donoke Beech Mein Sadiyose

Pyaarka Deep JalRahaHai"

I shall wait for you tomorrow at 4pm near 41st street in your area.

Yours Raja

I was eager for the next day. As soon as the sun rose, I wore blue TantSaree, blue bangles, blue earrings and red rose in the pony. My family members were surprised and well pleased to see a new look. Granny was suspicious about this sudden new change, as only we knew about 'Raja' in the fairytale.

My mind had beenconstantlyon the clock to see that it ticks 4 o'clock, for the first time the classes looked uninteresting! I got lost in myself like a sheep lost in a herd. I ran out of school at 3:30 p.m. to catch a tram and then human-pulled rickshaw to reach the 41^{st}street. I stopped the rickshaw at a distance and then walked.

I stood in the street looking dejected and decided to leave after 15 minutes of waiting. I heard a voice that took my breath

"TereHusn Ki Khaan To Main Dekh Hi Chukka Tha,

Aaj Teri AdaaonKaJalwaBhiDekhLiya,

Tum Sach Me BehadKhubsurat Ho,

AajKhudakaYehKarishmaBhiDekhLiya"

He held my hand and pulled me near his face to kiss. I pushed him and began to run back towards home. In his loud voice, he said

"Tujhse Main KitnaPyaar Karta Hoon,

Ye SirfAurSirf Mai Hi JantaHoon,

Tum Hi Ho MeriDil-ruba

AajMain Dil Se YehMaantaHoon"

I turned back and said, intezaarkarnamera (wait for me). He nodded his head in affirmation. I was swinging, jumping, picking leaves from the branches of trees on my way, laughing, yelling and singing. Granny was at the doorstep. I ran into the house with the signature shyness of mine and the life started to look beautiful!

Every moment of waiting was heavy and wait for 4 o'clock was like waiting for a birthday to come next year. The next day I made a prank of reaching half an hour late, he wasn't there. The prank and the wait of 30 minutes werefutile. While back home dejected, someone pulled my veil and I turned to see a little boy; the boy pulled my hand to lean down and whispered something into my ear. The child pointed to Raja,he was now at a distance. The child gave a peck and ran away. I ran to Raja to hug him. We were spotted kissing and cuddling by granny and mother. Mother slapped Raja and pulled my hand in anger towards home. All the family members gathered in the hall with numerous questions that were unanswerable. For the first time,the father raised his hand and caned me black

Second Heart

and blue. I was locked in the room with instructions from Dada (father) not to provide any food or water.

Later in the night, granny came with some food. I was crying, lying on the floor.

Granny: Othoshona, ektukheynao (Baby, get up, have some food)

Me: Kona (No). Amar raja k chai (I want Raja)

Granny: Shona, Raja Ekati Rupakatha Chilo, ektagolpo (Baby, Raja was a fairytale)

Me: (Crying loudly)

Granny: Ektukheynao Shona, tomar raja choleashbe (Have some food baby, you will get your Raja)

Me: Pratisruti? (Promise?)

Granny: Pratisruthi Shona (Promise Baby)

Granny sang a quiet, gentle song to send me to sleep. Later that night my family members decided to marry me to one of our relative within a week. Naina overheard this conversation and around five in the morning informed me about this through a peephole. I was broken down and shattered on hearing this. I was kept under strict vigilance in the house. No one was allowed to meet me from outside. I requested Naina to help me.

Me: Naina, I will die without Raja.

Naina: Didi (Sister), don't talk like this.

Me: Please take this letter to Raja.

Naina:	Do you really want me to do this?
Me:	You are my only hope. Please do that for me.
Naina:	Ok

Naina handed over the letter to Raja. Naina got a note back from Raja.

Me:	How is he?
Naina:	He waits for you every day at 4p.m.
Me:	Oh, why is this happening to me?
Naina:	He gave this note for you
Me:	I hurriedly opened to read

"TereKhamoshChehreKoDekhkar Mai Kya Kahun,

Ye Sab BayaanKarDetaHai,

IsmeChupaHarPehlu

Zindagi Mein SeekhaSabaqBayaanKarDetaHai"

Let's elope from this world to paint our new world. If your answer is 'yes', come to Howrah station tomorrow evening at the ticket counter.

Me:	Yes, Yes…
Naina:	Didi, what is it?
Me:	I showed the note to Naina.
Naina:	Didi, don't do such a thing. Dada will kill you and me.
Me:	Trust me, nothing will happen. This is my life; I would want to marry the one I love.

Second Heart

Naina: But..Didi..

Meanwhile, I went to the Dada and asked for forgiveness. Dada and others in the family were delighted to see that I am ready to marry their chosen one. I winked to Naina to signal this was a prank. I took all the money from the piggy bank and a pair of clothes to elope after the sunset. I took the route from the terrace, jumped to the neighboring building, and got down from the toilet pipe. Naina was at the terrace to see me leave with a fear of the outcome. I reached Howrah station; Raja was next to the ticket counter.

Me: Which is the train? Where are we going?

Raja: We are not going by rail.

Me: Then….

Raja: Your family will catch us in case we go by bullock cart (passenger express). I have arranged a car to leave for Delhi.

Me: Why Delhi?

Raja: I shall tell you about it as we move.

Me: Ok

I felt a bout of the jitters, travelling with an unfamiliar person. Is this a blind love? Countless such questions were running through my minduntil we reached Delhi. We reached there in the wee hours.

Me: What next?

Raja: We shall stay here for a week and take the sea route to the Middle East.

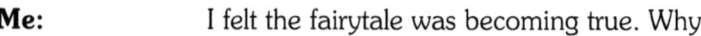

Me:	I felt the fairytale was becoming true. Why are we going there?
Raja:	I work there.
Me:	We went to one of his friends places. The place was located in a very closed locality. I didn't want to question all these small things, as we were there for a short time.

Someone greeted him in a way I did not know anything. After some breakfast, I was with Raja at the roof of the house.

Me:	Raja, why did you greet that way?
Raja:	That's the way it's greeted.
Me:	What's your full name?
Raja:	Raja Ismail
Me:	Are you ....?
Raja:	Yes
Me:	Oh God!
Raja:	(smiles)Why do you measure our love through religion?
Me:	Not that way, but ....
Raja:	We have a long journey ahead.

We went to Gujarat and took a ship to a far-off place in the Middle East. The huge Indian Ocean, open sky, stars, full moon, and a cold wind fascinated me during the nights and a bright sunshine during the day.

Second Heart

Me:	When will we get married?
Raja:	We are already!
Me:	When?
Raja:	The day we saw each other.
Me:	(smiles) I would like to be officially married to you.
Raja:	The Wide Ocean and the open sky are the witness. I accept you as my wife. Do you accept me as your husband?
Me:	(With Signature shyness) Yes.

We arrived at some town. There were two tall men who came to receive us. They spoke some language that I did notunderstand. I was afraid of their mighty built or looks which were no less than villains (UtpalDutt or Uttam Kumar) of Bengali movies. The street where the car moved had a unique atmosphere. The roads had the glitz and sophisticated nightlife. Many people have been out on the roads talking, buying and selling. We moved with our minimum baggage to a one-room house in the (last) third floor. I was about to get into the shower to freshen up; he pulled my veil (Towel) stuck to the body. That was the first time that someone touched my body. We made love that night. A feeling of a complete woman was getting generated.The fairytale looked true.

The house didn't have any ventilators further than the door; I could hear someone's prayer in the next door through the wall. As it got dark, I became anxious, as Raja didn't return. I fell asleep waiting for him. It may be past midnight; I heard a strong noise of someone banging the door. I went near the door with lit candle in hand. I heard Raja's voice, telling me to open the door. I saw Raja in a drunken state with a man at the door.

Me:	Are you drunk?
Raja:	Don't you see that?
Me:	(Crying)
Raja to man:	This is Maya, enjoy with her. She is yours.
Me:	What are you saying?
Me:	Raja pushed me inside. The man came into the house. Raja locked the door from outside.
Me to man:	Listen, I am his wife. It's sinful to do such a thing. Please don't come near me. I shall….
Man:	Husband? Your man has sold you. I am your client tonight. He gets girls like this every month. I have paid very high as you are fresh.
Me:	Please don't talk about all this. My Raja is not like that. He is tipsy and not aware of his act. Kindly leave home.

This was the first scream of help that was heard by none. I crashed to the ground in agony and was house arrested from 1987 onwards. I was provided with three meals a day with minimal medicines in case fell sick. I had become a puppet in the hands of cruel men and especially Raja. This betrayal had given birth to unbearable pain and anger. I had not seen bright

Second Heart

light for many years and was taken out only in the night to reach clients with eyes closed. The eyes were open only in the gloomy rooms with people guarding at the entrance. Every other day I was with someone else for next four years. The fear had engulfed in me so much; running away was a faraway dream. During these years, I survived only because of Peter.

I was broken, engulfed in fear; anger was highly intensified and hated men. There was one (Peter) in the neighboring house, often gave voice to talk.

Peter: Please talk to me. I cannot fully understand your pain, but would like to take some burden of yours.

Me: Go away. All you men are the same.

He would try to talk to me after each cry. It took me few months to get confidence that someone can hear my cry. He would read some prayers that could give me hope for life. He would try to learn few Bengali words and his pronunciations were funnier. I laughed at his pronunciation; the laugh that was hidden and buried deep down in my heart. I cried after this initial laugh as well. A new desire was born out of it.

Me: Peter, Peter

Peter: Yes, I am here

Me: I have a desire to see you

Peter: I shall find a way

Me: Please come soon

Peter: Yes, I shall

I tried hard to stop each man who came closer to me. They always overpowered me; only Peter heard my cry and all others were dead. I just wanted to resist every man who came for a minute pleasure. In these diminutive battles ofresistance, I hit Peter's head accidentally assuming him to be another man.

Me: Sorry Peter. I thought you were….

Peter: That's fine. I can understand your pain.

Me: You might have paid a lot to have an entry.

Peter: That's not important. Don't worry about it.

Me: Do you also want to…?

(Peter slapped me angrily. He apologized for being harsh.)

Me: For the first time, someone slapped for a good thing.

We had a heartfelt talk; while he left in the morning I gave him thanks. I asked him to come back soon. He couldn't come every alternate day because that would lead to suspicion in thosewho are associatedwith selling me each day. I even didn't know if Raja was aware about my condition. Even if he knew, what's the point?

Peter would read scriptures and I would hear through the wall during daytime. While Peter was with me one evening I had a severe headache, pain in the chest and breathlessness. He couldn't take me outside, as they would kill both. Peter called a Doctor Yassin to get her advice. With her advice, he tried a few thingsduring the next visit that could help me a temporarily relief. He was concerned about my ailing health. Peter got Dr. Yassin to his home; through the wall, she would speak to me to understand the issue. She just wanted to get some blood and urine samples to test and find evidence before any recommendation. The entire situation was challenging for us. Dr. Yassin knew that the people in human trafficking are powerful and can go to any extent that would risk my life. I also didn't have a visa and documents to get out of this country easily. Even if legal authorities are approached, bribery can hinder and the threat of life is larger. Peter and Dr. Yassin gave me a silver lining of hope that they would find a way to help me.

Dr. Yassin asked me few questions about the symptoms. I used to get swelling on my face in the early mornings, which I used to attribute to the fact that I was not getting proper sleep. I used to have blood in the urine often, which I would ignore. All this made Yassin apprehensive of some disease of kidneys. She got in touch with some of her colleagues in the West. Dr. Yassin told that she would be unable to help me entirely since it requires an expert to deal with this but said she would give it a try.

Peter came to me as a client during next week carrying two alcohol bottles. I was surprised with this behavior.

Me: Peter, you have become like other men.

Peter: What's the matter?

Me: What's this? Two bottles of ….

Peter: Stay quiet for a while. Dr. Yassin, are you there?

Me:	What is she doing at your place now?
Peter:	Please wait for a moment.
Dr. Yassin:	Peter, I hope you had enough practice with a syringe to get blood sample.
Peter:	I hope so.
Peter:	Listen....By the way, what's your name?
Me:	Maya, first time a client is asking my name.
Peter:	Alright, by the way, don't call me as a client. I don't like it. Anyway, I never took someone's blood. Please forgive me if it pains.
Me:	It may not be as painful as the pain I am undergoing.
Peter:	No emotional stuff, Oh! I am sorry.

Peter had carried small vials in the alcohol bottles to collect the samples of blood and urine. He carried syringessaying that he will take drugs later in the night to the people who send clients to me. I was getting touched by Peter's and Yassin's act. Hope was getting strengthened.

The samples of blood and urine, which Peter and Yassin collected, were sent to a doctor friend of hers in the far West. I was told to have a kidney disease; something called PIGN, which usually recovers completely if,given proper treatment. I was fortunate enough to get some medicines from Yassin to control my blood pressure during this episode. The whole process of getting my readings (report) and treatment was

Second Heart

tedious, but still Yassin took it as a challenge. She was in continuous touch with her friend from far West and finally I started to recover. My kidneys recovered and over a period of two to three months I was alright.

Yassin told me that there are certain kidney diseases, which are due to some minor infections that we ignore. I did have a skin infection, but could not do much about it.

I got accustomed to spend a great deal of time with them. She would tell me stories of patients, which made me, feel sometimes that there werethose who had much more pain than me. Both of them would take some time out of their work; play with me being on other part of the wall. I would let them know the stories narrated by Granny and sing Bengali songs gently. We had created a world that had only a wall in between us. Only nights looked harder to pass through many a time.

It was now overfour years; I got a desire to get back home. I cried for hours and Peter's call went overheard. Peter and Yassin were worried.

Me: Peter, Yassin.... I want to get back home. Help me get out of this hell.

Peter: We are listening....

Me: Please do something soon. I can't live like this.

Peter: Maya, we shall figure out a way. You trust us, right?

Me: Yes, I have only you both to trust.

Peter: Nope, you have three.

Me:	Three?
Peter:	God (Hope)
Me:	Yes
Peter:	Now smile and laugh, Baby

We began to laugh after hearing the word Baby, as only Granny addressed me. I felt as if, God has favored me. Peter and Yassin kept talking to me often to explain the challenges they have to face to rescue me out of this town. Yassin plotted a plan to lure the men seated at the entrance through drink and followed by attracting them to have fun with her and her friends. I was very afraid in case she is caught in this act. She would become a victim like me or face death. She hired a couple of people those were in flesh trading to lure these men. As Peter was the client for that day, he found anapproach to escape. Although we were successful, we couldn't get out of the town as a vehicle hit Peter on the runway. Yassin took us to her house to provide us with shelter and treat him. He took a few days to recover. Peter and I couldn't come out, as people were in search of us. Since he was also found missing from his house and this made people suspicious.

Yassin arranged for a boat to escape from the town and reach the nearest harbor. She felt apologetic for being unable to help more than this. Peter and I left Yassin's house after midnight to the neighboring seashore to get into the boat. As I sat in the boat, Peter was still on the shore. I asked him to get into the boat, but he denied. He just wanted to stay back in the town, as it's his place. He took a promise from me to begin a new life. He requested the boatman to sail as quickly as possible. The distance from Peter was getting larger; I heard a pistol shot noise. I saw Peter fall on the ground. His sacrifice healed all the pain I had faced until.

I sat in the boat with a heavy heart. The boat reached a harbor; according to Yassin's instructions I reached one of the harbors of my country. Before I got down from the boat, the boatman gave me a gift that was wrapped in the paper. There was a woolen woven jacket given by Yassin and Peter with 'Shalom' written on it. I reached Calcutta after countless days of struggle by overcoming people's wrong motives. I fought against those odds through Peter and Yassin's scriptures. It was more than five years since I left this city. With a lot of excitement to see all the family members, I ran towards home. As I approached home, the tears became uncontrollable. As soon as, I knocked on the door. Dada opened it. Watching me, he shut the door immediately. I kept knocking saying, Dada its Maya. Please forgive me Dada. I wish to live with you all. Mother was in tears stood near the window and Naina came running to open the door, but Dada pulled her back. I began to scream and call Dida 'see your Shona has come. Don't you want to talk to me Dida?'

Mother: Maya, Granny is no more. She had a heart attack after you left the home.

Me: I am so sorry. Please forgive me.

Mother: Maya, go back to the place from where you came. (Mother shuts the window)

I walked back from home with sorrow and regret. Now I am seated at the railway station with tears rolling through cheeks with two options that run through my mind in this heavy monsoon. A train will arrive in which Raja will get down to take me back to the same world or do I listen to Peter and Yassin's Shalom message?

Doctor's diary:

Certain kidney diseases can occur with seemingly minor infections, which we are inclined to ignore. If neglected it can even become catastrophic in some cases and can lead to severe renal failure. Who would be that unlucky person is hard to predict. Skin infections and throat infections, which are very common and minor and self-limiting many times, but they can rarely lead to renal failure. Loose stools can cause dehydration and lead to kidney failure. All these are very common infections and seemingly insignificant can cause renal failure if neglected.

* * *

Thank you for reading our book. If you enjoyed it, won't you please take a moment to leave us a review at your favorite retailer?

Thanks,

Dr. Sandeep Huilgol

Santosh Avvannavar

Second Heart

Dr. Sandeep Huilgol : Sandeep did his medical schooling from Karnataka Institute of Medical Sciences, Hubli and he underwent his medical training at Mallya Hospital a leading super specialty hospital in Bengaluru. During his medical training, he developed a special interest in nephrology, which deals with kidney diseases. After having spent a year in the Nephrology department to complete his Masters at the University of Sheffield, United Kingdom he returned back to India to undergo further training in Nephrology and transplantation at Narayana Hrudayalaya, Bangalore.

He has published articles on kidney diseases in National daily and an international magazine apart from academic publications and presentations. He is also part of an initiative, a journal that is trying to create a platform for the resident to publish academic articles. During his Nephrology training, he has come across many patients with various problems other than medical that were more troublesome than kidney diseases. This prompted him to come up with an idea to create awareness among the general public about the matterand he has given several talks to achieve this objective with which he is not satisfied yet and aims to reach a larger audience in future.

Santosh Avvannavar: Santosh started his career as a consultant and Soft Skills Trainer. He did his college education from NITK, Surathkal. He functioned as a researcher at University of Eindhoven, University of Twente and Indian Institute of Science, Bangalore. He was also the Placement President, while he was working at IISc, Bangalore. He has over 25 publications of mostly research documents that have found their place in National & International Journals. Also, he has done 16 conference papers and regularly functions as a writer of different articles for a national and worldwide daily paper.

He is an advisorfor different organizations. Throughout his personal time he composes his thoughts on a website, namely www.amritafoundation.wordpress.com and ventures into fiction writing. He delivered seminars and training to more than 33,000 people in India and abroad over the span of 7 years.

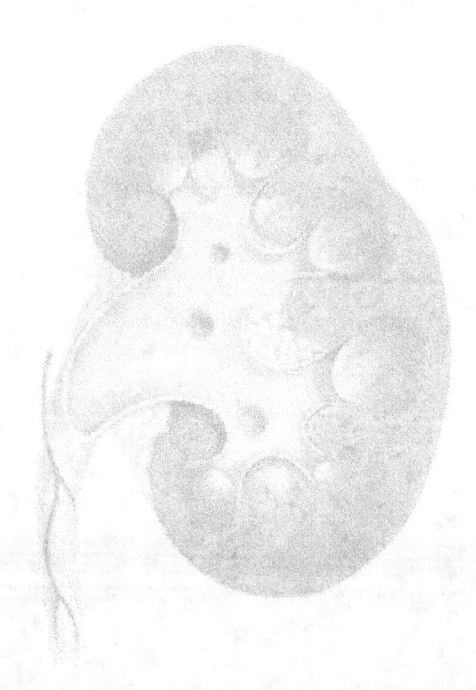

www.ingramcontent.com/pod-product-compliance
Lightning Source LLC
Chambersburg PA
CBHW071255170526
45165CB00003B/1357